Mind Power

Strategies On How To Avoid Distraction And Keep Your Concentration

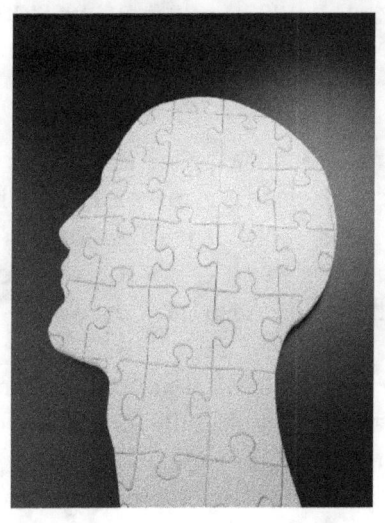

By
Fhilcar Faunillan

Fhilcar Faunillan

The information provided herein is stated to be truthful and consistent, in that any liability, in terms of inattention or otherwise, by any usage or abuse of any policies, processes, or directions contained within is the solitary and utter responsibility of the recipient reader. Under no circumstances will any legal responsibility or blame be held against the publisher for any reparation, damages, or monetary loss due to the information herein, either directly or indirectly.

Respective authors own all copyrights not held by the publisher.

The information herein is offered for informational purposes solely, and is universal as so. The presentation of the information is without contract or any type of guarantee assurance.

The trademarks that are used are without any consent, and the publication of the trademark is without permission or backing by the trademark owner. All trademarks and brands within this book are for clarifying purposes only and are the owned by the owners themselves, not affiliated with this document.

Table of Contents

INTRODUCTION

I want to thank you and congratulate you for downloading the book, *"Mind Power: Strategies on How to Avoid Distraction and Keep Your Concentration"*.

To start off, ask yourself the following questions:

Do you often find your mind wandering? Do you ever find it hard to pay attention to something a long stretch of time? Do you jump from one task to another? Do you find it hard to accomplish tasks, even simple ones, in one sitting?

Perhaps you have not yet discovered your mind's power or ability to ignore distractions and focus on important tasks. Everything around us may have their ways of getting into our nerves and into our minds. These distractions keep our brains off from working to their full potential. But our brain can still fend for itself by knowing how to concentrate. This mind power can bust off distractions that keep us from being productive and this mind power can be practiced, developed, and mastered.

Mind power of concentration is having the ability to focus on a task with full on attention. The more we can concentrate, the more we can finish tasks with good quality and efficiency. Concentration is an important source of human productivity. Without it, we would end up switching from one task to another without really getting anything done.

The benefits of concentration will be applicable to almost all aspects in your life. From your occupation, to your relationships with other people, and to yourself as well. Your concentration will keep you connected with all these aspects and will keep you living in the now, making you more emotionally, physically, and mentally healthy.

In this book, you will learn the secrets of your mind and its power of concentration. Benefits of this power of mind will also be discussed in this book, as well as the different kinds of distractions that you should be able to warn yourself with. Techniques in enhancing your power of mind in concentration will also be given in this book. Different exercises on concentration and self-regulation will help you expand your ability to focus.

Discover the capabilities of your own mind and experience all the benefits that your brain's full potential can give you. Begin by knowing what your mind is capable of and practice its capabilities to develop it fully. Make use of the contents of this book to find and tap on your mind power and keep your mind off all the distractions and connect on being able to concentrate.

Thanks again for downloading this book, I hope you enjoy it!

Chapter 1- Discovering The Mind's Power

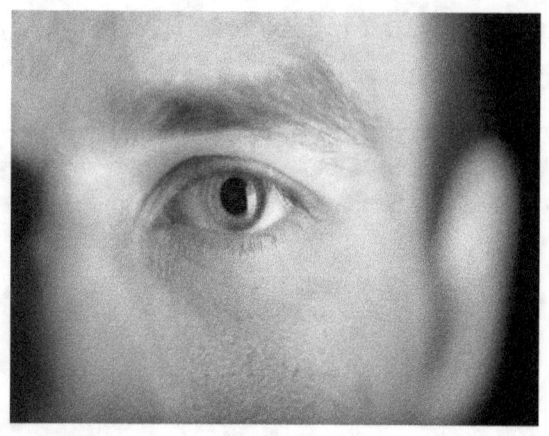

Swami Vivekananda, in his words has said...
"Mind powers are like the rays of the sun. When concentrated, they will illumine."

The Mind as an Energy Source

The Mind Over Matter theory is not a busted myth. Over the years, science has proved our thoughts to have power over our body, that if we regulate them, we can regulate our body as well. These thoughts may have physical manifestations that can affect our behaviors as well.

One of the major discoveries of science on this theory is of the Placebo drug which is a dummy drug that is harmless and basically just made of sugar that is only meant to make the patient believe that he or she is taking medication for his or her illness.

This drug has worked for depression and other body pains, reducing symptoms and reducing stress. Just the thought of these patients that they were taking drugs to cure their illnesses, had their brains anticipating the successful effect of these drugs which made their bodies respond in such a way that it mimicked wellness. Using PET scanners and MRIs, science took the step further into explaining how the brain works with the placebo. With the dummy drug, the thinking of the patient changes the chemistry in the brain causing the brain to react in physical ways as well. These chemical changes translated into responses by the body itself.

This discovery gives us the idea that the brain is capable of doing things that extends over our expectations.

Mind Power of Concentration

One of the important aspects and purposes of human life is to accomplish tasks effectively and efficiently and this duty needs a mind power.

Perhaps you have tried being so engrossed in a book that you were reading or a movie that you were watching, that everything else around you just seemed to blur into a background that you were not totally aware of. That was your brain concentrating. This is our brain's ability to direct or focus our attention on whatever we intend to and withdraw from focus when we want to, as well. Concentrating is one of the brain abilities that can be aided by the power of the mind and the theory of mind over matter.

But you have probably also have had your mind elsewhere while you were in a middle of a conversation or meeting. Perhaps you have tried reading an entire paragraph when you finally asked yourself what you have just read. It happens. Attention is a limited source and concentrating is quite of a challenge. Most of the time we seem to mindlessly wander elsewhere.

The particular area in our brain responsible for the ability to focus or pay attention is the lateral prefrontal cortex. The neurons in this area interact with each other in order to filter the information that they get from the environment through the visual sense.

They sift off the distraction from the information making concentration more effective and efficient.

We actually all have the ability to concentrate, that is, when we exert effort and time into doing it. Which means that sometimes we really cannot do so, especially with all the countless distractions around us. Mental concentration needs mental effort. And mental effort needs practice.

Our brains need to practice concentration strategies in order to be able to focus well. This full development of the ability to concentrate would not happen in a blink of an eye nor would it happen overnight. Our brains need to get exposed to these strategies of concentrating in order to channel attention effectively and more efficiently but it will take weeks and months. So you just have to be patient with yourself and do not give up.

Attention is only a limited source at first, but with constant practice and perseverance, it can be a limitless source of power in accomplishing many tasks successfully.

All these weeks and months of practice would not go in vain as you will need great concentration in doing so many things — from cooking, to driving, to studying, to working, and to many more activities in our day to day lives. It is an applicable practice to almost any aspect of our lives so devoting time, energy, and effort into mastering it is not a pointless matter.

We only use up a small percentage of our brain every single day that we are not really aware of its full potential and ability when we use it well. Mind power is one of the strongest and most effective ways to get you to do things well. This power mainly involves our thoughts.

Knowing that these are our thoughts gives us the key to develop this power well if only we watch and take control of these thoughts. These will shape and drive us as a person and will affect many aspects of our lives. So it is a necessary ability to be able to concentrate and avoid distractions.

Chapter 2 - Benefits Of Having The Power

Over Your Own Mind

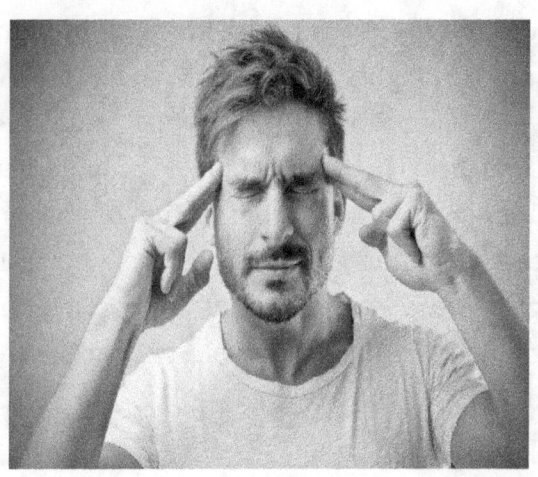

Before you engage with the strategies to keep your concentration strong and unwavering, know what you can get from them. The benefits of mind power can extend across different aspects of your life — from the most difficult task that you have to accomplish, down to the easiest one. The more you have power

17

over your own mind, the more you can concentrate and experience these benefits.

1.   Clarity of Thoughts

The ability to have control over your mind thoughts means that you can free your mind of useless and negative thoughts. These thoughts will only bother and distract you from doing important tasks. Getting rid of these thoughts can give you a peace of mind and a clarity of thoughts making you able to think more clearly.

2.   Better Memory

Because you can free your mind of all the unnecessary thoughts, you can already pay more attention to more useful information. The absence of these distractions lets your brain absorb these more necessary information better, which means that they could be retained for a longer time, even more efficiently.

3.   Increased Self-Confidence

Our mind power's concentration gives us the ability to dwell on ourselves. However, with proper self-introspection we can objectively see ourselves as people with flaws and good qualities. The more we know about these things, the more we know our limits. We improve our self-efficacy, further developing the confidence that we have for ourselves.

4.   Efficient Comprehension

With the absence of other thoughts that keep you distracted, you can focus more on processing information. The more attention you pay to something, the more you can process it quickly and more effectively.

5.   Happiness and Improved Mood

Another advantage of being able to have power over your own mind is imposing a positive emotion on yourself. This allows you to de-stress or reduce the stress hormone level in your body called the cortisol. When you are able to concentrate, your mind is of proper condition to think of more positive things instead of ruminating problems and worries. So you feel off of burdens, lowering your risks of having depression.

6.   Improved Emotional Regulation
Concentration allows you to have a more positive mind and an approach-oriented emotional state. This means that you improve your will and ability to face the real world and conquer your own problems rather than withdrawing from them.

7.   Increased Productivity
The ability to focus on a certain task for a long time allows you to become more productive. Concentration gives you lesser tendency to switch from one task to another that you end up without a finished output. More so, because you are

able to give your hundred percent attention to the task, you are also giving importance to the state and perfection of the output, considering that attention will never draw down the output's quality. With concentration you improve your performance: both on productivity and output quality.

8.   More Neural Connections

Mind power does not only involve behavioral evidence. It also goes down to the neural level in the brain. Constant concentration practice allows your brain to have more and stronger connections that make processing more efficient. Which makes you able to switch task simultaneously of one another and still pay attention to these tasks that is if the ability to concentrate has been developed well already.

9.   Improved Creative Abilities

Concentration allows our minds to formulate creative and innovative ideas. Ignoring distractions can make our brain work more on what it is supposed to. If you are meant to create a design or art, it is best to get drawn into the moment to have a better feel of your art.

10.   Safety and Security

When you are not really paying any attention with what you are doing, chances are, your mind will let important safety precautions slip away and with that, you might end up in an accident. You may have heard of countless road accidents due to multitasking while driving. This lack of concentration can cause far more harm than you could ever even think of. Imagine your mind wandering while you are ironing your clothes. The more it wanders, the more your clothes burn. Giving your full attention to your tasks allows you to avoid unwanted mishaps that may further cause harm.

Chapter 3 - Developing Your Mind Power

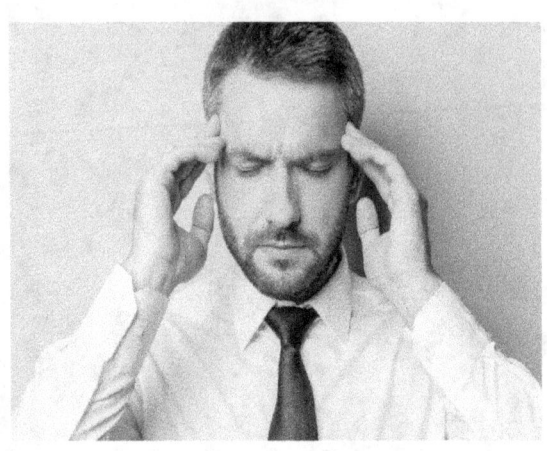

The Tilopa, Tibet said that...
"In the beginning, the meditator feels like his mind is tumbling like a river falling through a ravine; then, it flows slowly like the gently meandering River Ganges; and lastly, the river becomes one with the great vast Ocean, where the Lights of Son which is referred to as the self along with Mother or the ground of being, merge into one."

Mind Power

If the benefits of the mind power of concentration have convinced you, you might ask yourself of how your brain develops into its powerful state.

Developing your mind power is pretty much like developing your physical strength. Doing so takes a lot of patience, perseverance, and practice. But all of these efforts will pay off once your mind power has been fully developed. Then, it will be easy for you to shun distractions and devote more attention on accomplishing your tasks.

According to classic spiritual literature, your mind power concentration goes through three major stages: encompassing the ability to get distracted easily, to a gradual improvement on paying attention, to being as one with the object of concentration.

The development begins merely by being able to hold your focus momentarily on a task. Distractions will steal your attention every once in a while and completing a task may take longer than when you really dwell attention, time, and effort on it. In this first stage, your attention will gradually be sustained. Although it starts off with momentary concentration, the more you engage in it, the more it strengthens. So if at first you can thoroughly do something for seven straight breaths, the next thing you know you are indulged in a task for 21 straight breaths, up to 108 breaths or longer without ever losing your focus. So, there goes the progress.

The second stage is when your concentration can be sufficiently stable that you can no longer lose your focus, even with the occasional distractions and temptations coming. You develop a more profound relationship with the object of your focus that your brain does not stray away from it so easily anymore. By this time, you can experience a sense of connectedness as well as a sense of flow between you and the object of your concentration.

In the third stage, your mind power becomes so powerful that it will extend farther than just a connectedness but of a communion between you and the object of concentration. This is when the mind fully absorbs the task or subject of concentration that it engages in a unification with it and completely ignores distractions. By this time, more than just restricting yourself of all the distractions, you feel more oneness with the object which makes the focus stronger.

With a fully developed concentration, you may always be able to access your mind power in whatever task you may be doing. The ability to ignore distractions is not an easy feat, but with patience, perseverance, and practice, accessing the mind power's full potential is not an impossible venture.

Chapter 4 - Concentration Killers

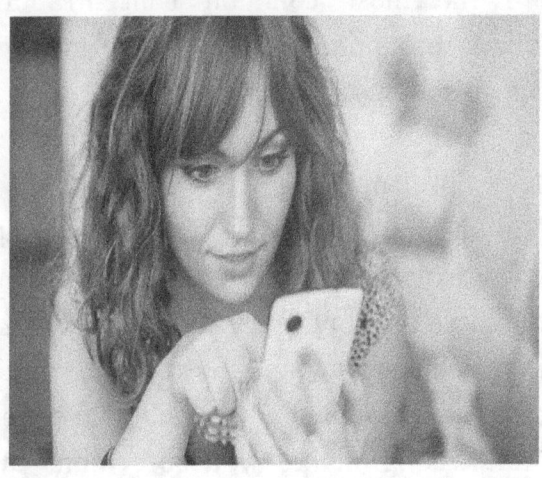

Concentration killers or distractions may come in different forms and degrees from either internal or external sources. They may get to you or you can choose to get them out of your way so you can accomplish your tasks. Before you get to do that, you have to be able to familiarize yourself with these concentration killers so that the next time you encounter them, you can mentally alert yourself to avoid them and swiftly note that you have to swerve to a more productive way. These are the most common concentration killers that hinder you from ever getting things done:

1.   Multitasking

Multitasking gives you the illusion that you are doing two, or even more, things at the same time but really, all you are doing is switching from one task to another, and to another, and not getting anything done. Multitasking makes you lose time by shifting to different tasks that you never really accomplish anything, or if you do, the quality of the outputs of these tasks will be at risk. Multitasking divides your attention as you shift from one work to another. And this does not really work especially when the tasks being done are complicated and high-priority ones. It is okay to talk on the phone while doodling but it is a different story when you are cooking while ironing your clothes.

Multitasking is only possible on easy tasks that you have already mastered really well but other than that, it is a huge cause of death of your concentration.

2.   Lack of Interest

If you do not want to do something, almost everything can distract you from doing it. Perhaps you have tried studying for a class that never sparked your interest, so you find staring at a wall even more interesting than checking your textbook. Boredom can take all of your ability to focus on doing a task, making your more prone to giving in to distractions. This lack of interest can translate to lack of action as well. So, when you know that something does not interest you well enough, prepare yourself for a struggle in finishing this task.

3.   Worrying and other negative mental thoughts

Our thoughts can hold so much power over us that when we are internally distracted by them, they can control and compel us from paying attention to other things. You may have experienced worrying about an upcoming exam, the effect of something that you said, or even about having no money at all. These thoughts can cloud our heads that most of the time, they are all we can think about. They then occupy the spaces in our brain that should be dedicated to doing something more productive so instead of acting on more important matters, we sit there mentally bothered and physically paralyzed.

4.   Electronic Gadgets
Our phones beep and, as if it is an automatic response, we grab them and reply immediately. We pick up distraction and even hold them close. All these instant messages, texts, and emails give us the need to reply as soon as we get

them that we stop every once in a while with what we are doing to attend to these messages. With our attention divided between our task and the call of these electronic gadgets, we never really can give our full concentration in accomplishing what is needed.

5.   Internet

It may always be a struggle to use the internet when you are supposed to finish a task. You may find yourself working yourself for 5 minutes and the next thing you know, you are scrolling down Facebook and Twitter for the next hour or so. The easy way of multitasking in the internet makes it a vulnerable place to give in to distractions.

6.   Fatigue

Fatigue is our whole system's number one enemy. When you are so tired that you feel like you are just floating through the entire day waiting for the sun to set, you will find it hard to pay attention to anything trivial. Lack of sleep may impair attention, short-term memory, and other mental functions.

7.   Side Effect of Drugs and other Medical Conditions

Poor concentration may also be caused by certain medical conditions like ADHD, sleep apnea, depression, anemia, thyroid disease. You might want to consult your doctor or psychiatrist for these medical issues if you ever start to experience the symptoms.

8.   Noise

Noisy places take away your attention to stimuli that are not necessary. Instead of working on your task, your brain is distracted by the unnecessary and disturbing sounds. Your attention splits that you cannot thoroughly focus on your supposed task.

Chapter 5 - The Distracted Mind

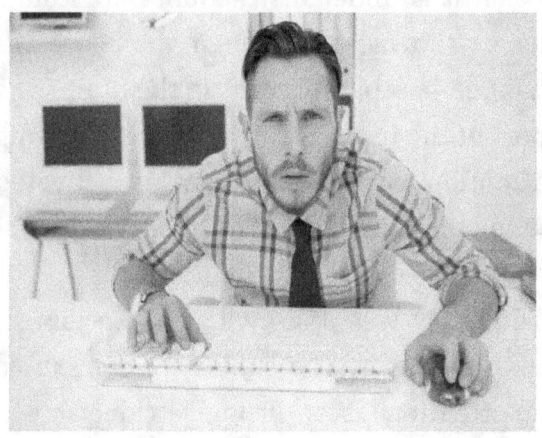

Thoughts may enter our minds with or without our own conviction. When we do not take control over these intrusive thoughts, they can cloud up our heads and keep us from focusing on more important matters.

A distracted mind can eat up so much of your time that could have been dedicated to productivity instead.

New research studies have shown how the brain works when it concentrates and when it is under distraction. And results have shown that the two processes happen in separate areas in the brain. One part of the brain is responsible for paying attention and another part is activated when the senses are distracted.

The study was done with an experiment with monkeys. The subjects were shown an attention tester through a video screen for an apple juice as a reward. They were meant to concentrate and pick out a certain object on the screen to focus their attention on—say a red box leaning on the left side of the screen.

However, flashes of attention grabbers are shown in the middle of the experiment. When the monkeys voluntarily concentrated on certain parts, an activation in the frontal area of their brain called the prefrontal cortex showed high levels of activity. When the attention grabbers appeared, the levels of activity was high on the back part of the brain or the parietal cortex.

Now that we know and understand how concentrating and distracting works in our brains, we realize how we can handle them. Moreover, knowing that these processes are independent of one another in terms of certain brain area activity, we can raise the possibility of working on them both independently — by improving concentration and reducing distraction.

Chapter 6 - Self-Regulation Strategies

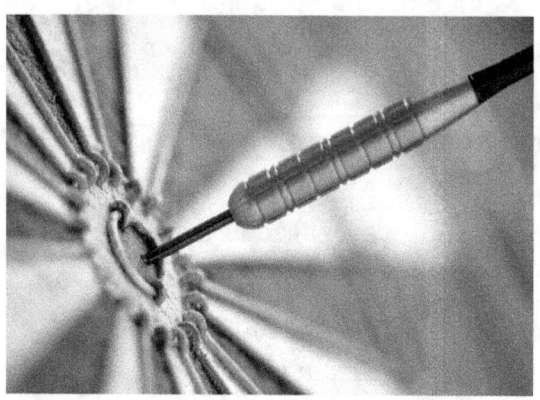

Concentration needs two of our major abilities: to exclude and to focus. These two abilities can both be accessed only with great self-regulation. Concentration is the strength of the mind that allows us to direct our attention towards something, as well as withdraw our attention when we want and need to. But with all the distractions and concentration killers around us, we often find it hard to devote all of our attention on a single task until it gets finished. Oftentimes, we find ourselves daydreaming in the middle of working, or scrolling down different social media sites for an hour when we promised ourselves we would only have a 5-minute study break.

Telling ourselves to stop and work is a whole lot harder than we think which is why it is also best to learn self-regulatory techniques in order to teach ourselves when to start working and stop procrastinating.

When the self is not under control, we are more vulnerable to distractions and temptations. Our appetites, mood swings, and impulses may get the best of us. Our weak self-guiding faculties may mean poor concentration as we care not able to control ourselves on what to focus on. An untrained mind and impulsive actions are not a good combination for concentration. Learn these self-regulation strategies in order for you to take direct action on your concentration.

1.   Be Here Now

When you notice that your mind starts to tick off elsewhere, remind yourself these three words: "Be here now!" You may use these words to police you from wandering off of your task and get you back on track.

2.   Learn From the Spider

When you allow a tuning fork to vibrate next to a spider web, the spider will initially look for the source of vibration. However, sooner or later, the spider learns that it is just you playing and not some bug that is ready to destroy the web. So, the spider goes back to building its web peacefully. If spiders can do it, then you can do it too. Take their weaving as you doing your own task. The ability of the spiders to shift their attention back to what they are doing, not minding distractions is the kind of concentration that your brain is also capable of. When you are in the middle of a class or work, and someone enters into the room. There may be a tendency for you to turn your head and look. But if you are in the middle of an important task, then looking may not be necessary and may only be a waste of your precious time. Control yourself not to give in to these kinds of distractions. Instead, pour your focus on what you should be doing. The next time someone enters into the room, train yourself not to look and continue working and learn from the spider's concentration.

3.   Worry Later

Set up some time for yourself to worry and think of all the thoughts that have been bothering you. Studies show that having a regular worry time decreases your intrusive worrying for 35% in a matter of four weeks. When you encounter a disturbing thought out of your scheduled worry time, brush it off by another self-regulation strategy (i.e., Be here now!) and tell yourself you will have time to worry about that later. Postpone intrusive worries for your scheduled worry time.

So, schedule a specific time of day for your worries. It could be at night, 7:00 to 7:30 pm or whatever time slot you prefer. Then think of the brushed worries that you had during the day. Most likely, you will be able to forget the worries that you were supposed to think of at that time. But other times, you will also remember them. When you remember these thoughts, you will have a much clearer head, which means that these worries may be able to find their match of solutions already.

4.   Wedging

Start off by a certain inertia in working on a certain task. After five minutes or so, ask yourself if you want to continue working or if you want to take a break. If you decide on the latter, make sure you have your kitchen timer on so you can immediately go back to work after taking a break. This way, you can give yourself some leisure, build your focus, and still be able to accomplish tasks gradually.

5.   Engage in a Reward System

Who does not want to see his or her payoff? Who does not want to celebrate over something that he or she have done successfully? Give yourself simple rewards when you finish your tasks. Match your rewards with how much effort your tasks need or how much you have exerted to do them. If you accomplish a heavy and important task, you may want to reward yourself with a good meal, a movie, an hour of internet surfing, or of anything with a heavier value for you. If tasks are only simple, you may just engage in simple rewards as well. You may allow yourself to read 5 pages of a certain book that you have always wanted to read or scroll down in Facebook for 10 minutes. Just make sure that the task and the reward match, so you it will also match your efforts. In rewarding yourself, it is important to note that you are not rewarding yourself for inadequate efforts exerted.

6.   Tally Lapses

While you are working on a certain task, set aside a piece of paper and pen, and tally the number of times that you have been distracted with something that is not part of your work. Record the duration of distraction as well. This way, you can keep track of how many times and how long you have wandered off of your supposed subject of concentration. This will give you an alarm if you have been slacking off way too much. This will also urge you to go back to work, focus, and be more productive.

One of the most difficult people to control, really, is ourselves. Sometimes we merely find it easy to brush off the things the warnings and alarms we remind ourselves of.

However, once you have conquered yourself in delegating effort on which tasks to focus on, you will find it easier to deal with the other factors of concentration (such as the environment and the diet). Most often than not, the self is the hardest person to fight against with. But with great effort and perseverance, conquering oneself is a fulfilling and satisfying task that can definitely translate to better and more useful results.

Chapter 7 - Concentration Strategies

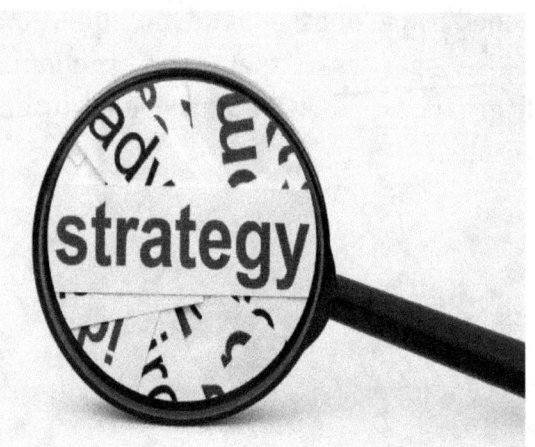

Different concentration killers may be addressed differently and specifically. If you recognize the hindrances you face to be under the stated concentration busters when you try to accomplish tasks then here are some techniques to battle them directly:

Multitasking

1.   *Schedule Your Tasks*

When you bulk in your tasks in one go, the tendency is that you would not know where to begin so you either do everything all at once or you end up not doing anything at all. But if you schedule all the things that you have to do in a day, with corresponding time for each task, then you would be able to know where to exert your effort on at a certain time of the day. For an additional tip, you may schedule your hardest and most effortful tasks in the morning when your willpower is at its peak. You may follow these tasks with simpler ones so the rest of your day could go smoothly.

2.   *Work One at a Time*

When you have already set your schedule, follow it and do one task after the other. You have made a schedule not to do the things all together but to give time for each of them. Keeping the tasks done separately will keep you focused on doing each one of them.

3.   Let Go Of Distractions

Some things will keep you doing more than one thing at a time. Your phone could be an instrument to never getting your tasks done because you always attend to it. So keep the phone away, turn the television off. Keep a clean space to avoid grabbing on distractions.

Mental Thoughts

1.   Let Thoughts Come and Go

Your thoughts can come like waves splashing on the shore, they may come and go as they are. How you analyze them will leave you with other mental thoughts and problems that were never really there in the first place. Practice letting these thoughts come and go. When you start to think about something, then allow it to enter your mind but do not give it any judgment or analysis, just let the thought be. Then, just as it came, let the thought go. This may be difficult at first but with constant practice, this will help you avoid worrying and other negative mental thoughts.

2. *Make Plans*

Keep a schedule on your weekly and daily plans. One of the reasons why people worry is that they do not really know what is going to happen next. Once you have laid out the things that you have to do in a month, in a week, and in a day, you know where you are heading. Keep a plan and have control over the happenings in your life. This way, you can worry less of what is going to happen next because you know that you are heading somewhere.

Fatigue

1. *Have a Regular Exercise*

One of the reasons why you cannot have a good quality of sleep is a disturbance in your health and well-being. Engaging in regular exercise and pairing it with a good and healthy diet will allow you to have a better quality of sleep at night.

2.   *Take Breaks*

Your brain and body can only work for a certain period of time. Without breaks in between, your system to crash in the long run. Give yourself a reasonable amount of time to rest in between doing tasks. Give yourself a breather. This way, the next time you work on your task, you will be more refreshed and thus, more productive. If you are familiar with the 'power nap' then you certainly know its significance especially in retention.

3.   *Look for Your "Prime Time"*

There will be a time in a day when you will be very productive, you can call that your "prime time". Find out if you work best early in the morning, or in the afternoon, or late at night then do your tasks during your prime time to avoid forcing your body to work so hard.

4.   *Listen to Your Body*

Your body will show signs that it is not doing well; so learn how to listen to it. When you are starting to get sick and feel more exhausted than usual, then you might need to consider taking a rest. Remember that your body is your capital in working, without it you will not be able to work your best so do not take your health for granted.

Lack of Interest

1.   *Reconnect*

Perhaps one of the reasons why you have lost your interest in doing a task is also the loss of its meaning. At some point in your task performance, you will forget why you have been doing it in the first place. All you have to do is rekindle your love for your task. You may ask yourself the reason why you had yourself into doing it in the first place. This may be a class you never really liked but ask yourself why you enrolled yourself into it. It may be because of your will to graduate. So hold yourself together and do it for a purpose.

2.   *Work Actively*

Admit it, there are tasks that never really spark your interest because they are plainly boring. But, you can spice them up by working on them actively. If you are studying on an interest-killer subject, you may want to talk to yourself while studying or use highlighters when taking down or rewriting notes. Make the task more fun and engaging for yourself so you can work on it for a few long hours.

3.   *Work With Someone*

You spend almost all your time with yourself that it may also get a little too boring. Working with someone adds spice on whatever task you are doing. If you need to focus on finishing a paper in class, grab a partner in a coffee shop and work on your paper. This added pressure will improve your task performance, making you more productive. Most people especially work best under pressure.

Electronic Gadgets

1.   *Turn Off Your Gadgets*

Nothing will keep on beeping if you just shut off your electronic gadgets. Lay it away from you and forget about their existence for a while. Work on your task without your phone or tab right beside you. Turn it off and place it away from you to avoid temptations. Try this and notice the changes.

Turn off Social Media Notifications on your Phone or Tab

If turning off your gadget may be too much for you, at least turn off the social media notifications that makes your phone beep every once in a while. Not knowing that someone commented on your post will keep you from asking yourself what that person has said. So, keep off from what these electronic gadgets can bring you by turning off their notifications.

2.   Do Not Work Near the Television

The nearer you are to the electronic gadget, the more vulnerable you become to it. So as much as possible, if you are working on an important task, stay away from electronic gadgets such as the television most especially that it can attract our sense of vision so easily and quickly.

Internet

1.   *Go for Minimal Tabs*
Open only tabs that are necessary for the task that you are doing. Avoid logging in to your social media accounts and other sites that will only distract you from your task. Go for minimal tabs and have maximum productivity.

2.   *Make Use of the Utilities*
Even the internet can help you keep off from its own distractions. Make use of different utilities such as Greasemonkey Script which you can use in Mozilla Firefox with Greasemonkey extension. In here you can utilize invisibility Cloak or Kiwi Cloak to block, for a predetermined time, sites that will kill your concentration. You can also use Time to Go. This will allow you to log into the concentration killer sites for only a certain amount of time. At least then, you know exactly where you will go back to.

3. *Turn off the Internet Connection*

If you cannot really hold your self-control, the best option for you is to just shut down your internet connection and work offline. Without the internet connection, you will not be tempted to log in to any site.

4. *Take a Distraction Time Off*

One of the reasons why you become unproductive and unable to focus is the overexertion of focus on a task for a lone time that the next time you look at it, it no longer makes sense to you. Take your time off and chill for a while. Have a break for 5 to 10 minutes. You may scroll through the different sites you considered distracting but make sure you can bring yourself to a halt when you know you already have to get back to work. Then so, work again. By this time, your brain is more refreshed and calmed down so your brain will have a more efficient and effective processing, allowing you to focus well.

Noise

1.   *Silent Spot*

Find yourself a perfect spot or hideout where you can work with minimal to no noise around. It may be in a café, in your room, or in your school library. Make yourself comfortable in that spot and start working and whacking on your task and you will surely be productive.

2.   *Make Your Own Playlist*

Our identification of what noise sounds like may still differ. Some prefer to work with soft music on the background while some consider rock songs like soft songs. Whatever your music preference may be, you can choose your songs and make your own working or studying playlist. Just make sure that you will not spend your time singing along to all the songs instead.

Chapter 8 - Concentration Exercises

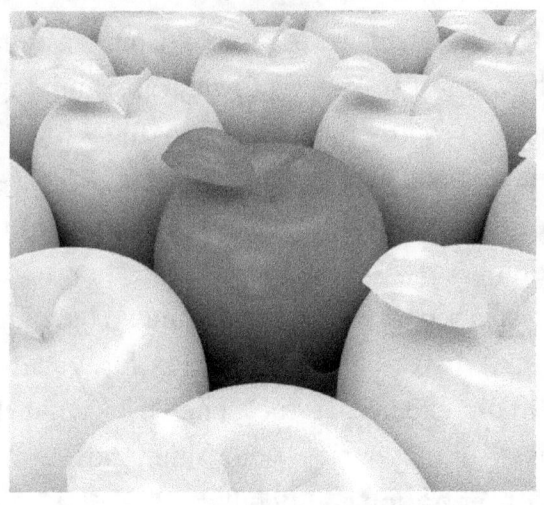

Just like a muscle, your mind power needs a lot of practice in order for it to reach its full potential of concentrating. Practicing this ability needs effort and patience for it to develop fully. Which is why you have to engage in some concentration exercises every day. In your daily schedule, set aside some time for exercising your concentration. You may try the different exercises as suggested in this chapter.

The following are sample exercises on how you can keep your neurons jumping and communicating, making more efficient pathways for thinking. These exercises will help you ease your way into doing tasks rather than respond to distractions every single time. You may want to try these strategies for you to finally experience the benefits of what it is like to develop your mind power of concentration ability fully:

1.   Counting Backwards

Count backwards starting from 100. Do this mentally and focus on thinking about the next number. If thoughts may come, let them drift away and go back to paying attention on the next number. You may also do a variation of this exercise by counting backwards by threes. Start by 100, 97, 94, so on, and so forth. You can also focus on counting backwards by fours, or by twos, or if you want, by prime or composite numbers as well.

2.   Word Focus

Think of a single word that inspires you. You may either say the word aloud or just keep it inside your head. If other thoughts may intrude, shift your attention back to the word and repeatedly say it out loud or just repeat it inside your head.

3.   Fruit Focus

Find any fruit and hold it in one hand. Feel the edges, the smoothness of the skin of the fruit, and smell its freshness. Focus your attention on the attributes of the fruit and if distracting thoughts may intrude, switch your attention immediately back to the fruit. Do this for at least 5 minutes.

4.   Whole Watch Way

Take a random object near you—whether it be a pen, a glass, or a fork. Look at the object's shape, color, and edges without verbalizing what you have observed. Dwell on the characteristics and properties of these objects. You may not know that there parts of them that you never really noticed. Spend at least 5 minutes of doing this exercise.

5.   Stay Still
Find a steady sitting position and make yourself comfortable. Focus your attention on keeping your body still and unmoving. If you do move, shift back into concentrating immediately. Do this for 5 minutes, at the very least. Then do it for 10 minutes, 15 minutes, and even more when you already can. Challenge yourself.

6.   Close-Open
Sit on a chair near a table and put your hands atop of it. Clench your fists and stretch your arms away from the table.

Slowly, open your firsts and look at your hands as it gradually extends its fingers. Open it really slowly and focus on its opening. Ignore any other thoughts other than the opening and stretching of your palm and fingers.

7.   Finding the Inner Flow

Find your inner flow through your mind power. Lay down on a comfortable position but avoid falling asleep. While laying down, imagine or visualize your blood moving through your veins all around your body. Focus on one part at a time, the shift to how it travels to another part. Do this for at least 5 minutes, then 10, until how far you can go. This will help you become more aware of your body's state.

8.   Mirror Trust

Stand in front of a mirror and draw or put two marks within your eye level in your reflection. Imagine this as another person's eyes. Imagine this other person as the very person whom you trust the most – he or she could be a friend, lover, parent, sibling, or anybody in your life. Focus on staring into the marks as if you are looking into the eyes of the very person you are imagining. If you find peace and comfort in this other person, chances are you will be more at ease and worry- free after doing this exercise. Sometimes, we just need to know and be reminded we are not alone in whatever problems we face. This exercise is for those who tend to worry too much that it already impedes their thinking.

9. Sifting Sounds

This exercise may be done in any place at any time. You just need your sense of hearing and your attention. You may stay in a busy street and sift sounds in the atmosphere. You may identify the sound of a certain car and focus on it for at least three to five minutes, then shift your attention to another sound. Or you may also stay in a coffee shop and distinguish sound sources as well. You may listen to the grinding of the coffee beans the shift to the sound of their café's soft music, then to the soft chatter of the people.

10. Word Count

Grab a book and count the words contained within a page mentally. Do not read or even analyze the words inside your head, just count. Proceed in doing this up to the next five pages. Do the counting as far as you can go. Challenge yourself. This may sound like an easy task but we know how we easily we can get distracted. This exercise will allow you to focus more even without verbalizing your thoughts.

Chapter 9 - Food For The Brain

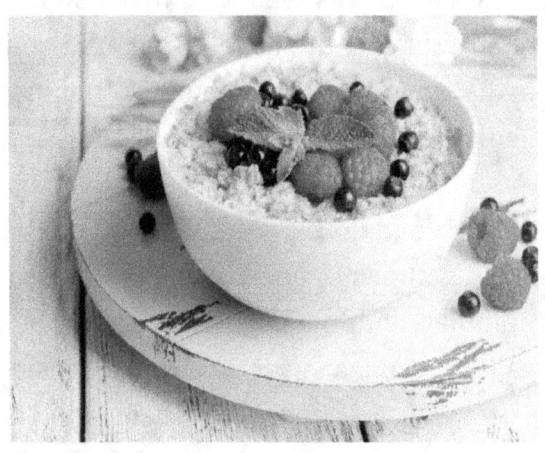

One of the factors that might affect your lack of concentration is poor nutrition. Not getting the right amount and proper sources of vitamins, minerals, and other nutrients can keep your brain from functioning well. Just imagine that your concentration is also quite similar to one important organ in your body that has to function every single day. You know that losing this organ can be very crippling. Which is why, like any other organ in the body, your mind, in order for it to concentrate effectively and efficiently, has to be fed with the proper and right amount of nutrients. Proper diet is recommended for better concentration.

Brain foods like the following are best for boosting your mind's ability to focus all throughout the day. So, add these up to your daily meals:

1.   Oatmeal

Breakfast is a very important meal of the day, most especially when you have a long day ahead of you. You need to kick your brain right in the spot by feeding it with the proper food. Oatmeal can be a great source of energy only with low caloric values. When you know you are up to a long list of tasks for the entire day, you definitely have to opt for a stomach-filling and satiating breakfast. Oatmeal can keep your fuller for longer hours which means you would not have to worry or even be bothered by a ranging stomach while you are working or trying to concentrate.

2.   Dark Chocolate

Dark chocolate in its right amount, which is one square serving, is enough to experience its benefits on your concentration. Dark chocolates can help your system produce more serotonin and endorphins. These are neurotransmitters that are associated with improved concentration. More so, its nutrients can also aid blood flow in the brain, making cognitive processes, including concentration, more efficient.

3.   Water

Dehydration leads to fatigue. When we are tired, we just want to get rid of every task that we have to do by getting it done without ever really exerting focus on it. Which is why they get done with poor quality. This fatigue impairs our ability to focus and accomplish tasks effectively.

Sometimes, the main cause of this tiredness is mainly because we are dehydrated. Drink lots of water to keep yourself running on enough fuel. With it, you tire less and do more instead.

4.   Blueberries

Blueberries are not only good for snacking but studies have shown that they are also memory boosters as they improve one's ability to concentrate and comprehend more.

5.   Salmon

Salmons contain high levels of omega-3 fatty acids which help the body rebuild cells, decrease cognitive functioning decline, and also strengthen the connections in your brain, most especially those that are related to concentration and memory. Salmon's protein which contains amino acids are those that help the brain develop sharpness and focus.

6.   Coffee

Coffee helps in the release of norepinephrine in the body. This is the neurotransmitter that tells your body to stay alert. Once it cues the body to stay on that state, it is capable of focusing for longer time duration already.

7.   Green Tea

Green tea contains the amino acid called the theanine. This amino acid has shown to improve mental sharpness and focus. Green tea also contains caffeine which helps in the release of norepinephrine, however, it is more natural to drink as compared to coffee as the latter may have adverse side effects in the long run.

8.   Beets

Beets have high levels of nitrate that can help dilate the blood vessels, increase blood flow in the system, and transport oxygen into the brain, thereby improving mental performance, including the ability to focus.

9.　Bananas

Bananas are very well known to be great potassium sources. Potassium is a mineral that is essential in keeping the nerves, heart, and most especially, the brain in their best shapes and functioning.

10.　Spinach

Spinach contains high levels of lutein, folate, and beta-carotene. All of these nutrients are known to be associated with preventing dementia—one of the cases when concentration is highly impaired. Spinach is a very good brain food and can easily be added as a garnish in different dishes.

11.　Eggs

Eggs are also loaded with enough omega-3 fatty acids that can help in **improving memory and positive mood. More so,**

they contain a compound named choline that can aid in keeping the cell membranes in the brain healthy.

12. Green Leafy Vegetables

Green leafy veggies are rich in fiber and many other nutrients that can sustain the energy level of the body. When the body has its optimal energy, it can work without being bothered by fatigue and worries, making the brain more engaging in concentrating.

13. Tomatoes

Tomatoes are rich in antioxidants that help the cells in the brain reduce inflammations, as well as improve blood flow and oxygen transport in the system. These can make the brain be in perfect state for its cognitive functioning, including concentrating.

14. Meat Dairy

Dairy from meat is good for the brain in little amounts. They are rich vitamins B6 and B12 that prevent memory and other brain problems from developing (such as Alzheimer's and dementia). However, consuming meat from dairy should be kept in moderate amount only.

15. Avocadoes

Avocadoes are rich in fiber which can aid in improving the blood flow in the body, allowing more efficient transportation of nutrients to the organs, including the brain. More so, avocadoes can also fill your stomach longer. So if you are preparing to work on something for a long time during the day, you can eat avocado before working on that task.

16. Flax Seeds

Flax seeds contain B-Vitamins, Omega-3 fatty acids, as well as fiber. All these nutrients and minerals are necessary for

73

mental clarity making one more able to concentrate or pay attention. You can have flax seeds grounded and sprinkled over your oats, salad, or cereal.

17.   Nuts

Nuts have high vitamin E content—associated with reduced tendency of cognitive performance as one ages. Munch on some nuts for snacks or throw them in as small ingredients in different dishes of which you prefer.

Dieting for the brain to be able to concentrate well is not exactly a very engaging task at first but when you think to yourself and commit to a lifestyle that treasures productivity, growth, development, and activity — engaging in a brain food diet would not be so hard to do. Much like self-regulation, engaging in a diet for the brain's ability to concentrate better requires dedication, commitment, and discipline. It will not be easy but it is not impossible.

Chapter 10 - Find A Home for Your Mind Power

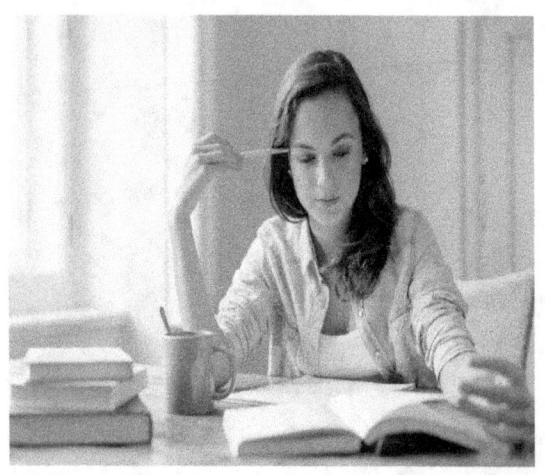

Sometimes the very thing that hinders you from performing really well does not entirely rely on your lack of discipline, rather, of the chaotic environment that you are in. One does not only have to master the self. Doing so would only be futile if one cannot master and control the environment for it to be more conducive for concentrating as well.

The following are tips on how you can create an atmosphere and situations that would be favorable for concentrating:

1. Find a quiet place

First things first, find yourself a perfect place to work at. You need to consider several aspects in choosing the place: Is it quiet here? Can I bring myself to keep myself motivated in here? Is it convenient?

When you choose a place, make sure that the aspects that you are looking for belong to the place. Sometimes it takes a lot of canvassing—you may experience hopping from coffee shop to another until you find the perfect one with affordable and tasty coffee, reliable internet connection, quiet atmosphere, and the perfect working ambiance. Also, you might hop from one public library to another until you find the one that is not too crowded and has the resources that you might need. In any way, find yourself your working or studying haven that can be conducive for your focus to work well.

2.   Prepare the stuff you will need

Do not bother yourself into thinking about something else while you are already in the middle of doing a task. Prepare all the stuff that you will need when you work or study. Pack up your laptop, notes, highlighters, pens, papers, and other whatnots and essentials. So when you need them, you do not have to waste time in looking for them and taking them into your workplace. Time is your most precious commodity when you concentrate.

3.   Find a constant working spot

Once you find the perfect spot, be a regular already. Finding that place to be encouraging of your motivation to keep on working will make you want to stay there. Do not be afraid to commit to this place, because the more you visit it to work at, the more your brain familiarizes the spot as a cue to get you working. Take this as a matter of conditioning your brain to work.

4.   Sit with a pen and paper

Studies have shown that keeping a pen and paper on one side of your working area will keep you closer to writing your tasks down, keeping yourself on track, and making yourself more immersed in you tasks. Take down notes even while you are working. The more tangible these notes are, the more they stick to you.

5.   Vary working or studying activities

Being repeatedly exposed to a stimulus makes it more and more boring. No matter how much you like a class, if it no longer poses a challenge on you, it is as good as an old rag. So, in order to kill this developing boredom vibe, learn how to vary your activities and tasks.

Perhaps you may schedule different tasks for different days of the week then switch them again after two weeks or so. If you also want you can also make your duty and study more interactive—even with just yourself. Do not bore yourself to death and find ways to make your object of concentration more interesting and entertaining.

6.   Keep temptations away

Get a hold of you environment by keeping yourself at a safe distance from all the temptations around you—electronic gadgets, other people, movies, TV series, internet, and more. You may also include this in your criteria in looking for the perfect spot to work at. One of the best ways to keep yourself productive is to stay away from all possible temptations that may just steal your attention.

Mind Power

Aside from the self and the diet, having the optimal environment for working is also a necessary aspect that one has to look at one when he or she wants to be productive by being able to pay attention to his or her tasks.

Finding the perfect spot cannot really happen overnight, not even in just one go. More so, controlling the environment for it to become more conducive for working is also a challenging task as you can never really get a hold of all the factors in the environment. Still, that does not restrict you from doing what you can on making a home for your mind power in its very own environment.

CONCLUSION

Thank you again for downloading this book!

Now that you have finally reached the last part of this book, be ready to ask yourself the same questions again:

Do you often find your mind wandering? Do you ever find it hard to pay attention to something a long stretch of time? Do you jump from one task to another? Do you find it hard to accomplish tasks, even simple ones, in one sitting?

With the help of this book, you should be able to proudly say that distractions no longer impede your productivity and that your focus is much more developed than when you started reading this book. And more so, in further time as you engage in the given exercises and techniques every single day.

Because we know that how we go on our day by day lives is affected by how well we can concentrate. Most of the time, it is an ability that we take for granted, which is why many people end up in accidents and poor output quality and performance. At the end of the day, we feel satisfied with all the things we have accomplished. That is, if we were able to devote enough focus into them just to get them done. If not, then we realize how important concentration is.

Concentration needs two important parts. One is the ability to dismiss unnecessary information, second is the ability to direct attention towards a more important task. These two parts mean that you need to be able to control yourself and several aspects of your environment in order to successfully focus on a task. Doing both is a challenging feat but not impossible.

In order to develop your mind power's concentration completely, you must engage religiously in practicing it. Start off by devoting time and effort in doing concentration exercises every single day. The benefits of this mind power will all be enough to pay for all the efforts that you put in when you practice paying attention. It is an investment that will surely grow and benefit the different aspects in your life — from personal to social facets.

The techniques provided in this book are simple and very easy to do. You just need a few simple items that you can easily find around you. You may even be able to make variations out of the given techniques just as long as you keep its objective of developing one's concentration.

At the end of this course, you should be able to allocate some time to do these exercises and improve your concentration. Find out the capabilities of your own mind and how far it could take you when it knows how to pay full attention. Rest assured that the advantages will be of a good reap for you.

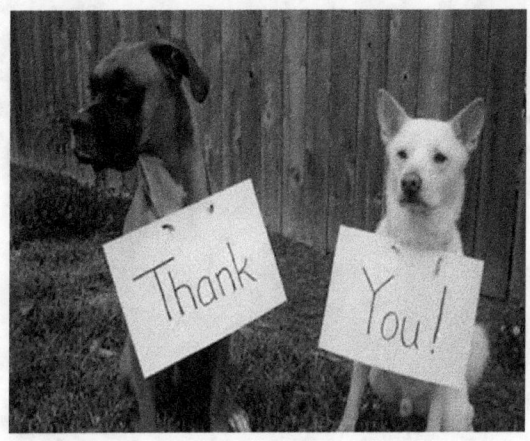

Finally, if you enjoyed this book, then I'd like to ask you for a favor, would you be kind enough to leave a review for this book on Amazon? It'd be greatly appreciated!

Click here to leave a review for this book on Amazon!

Thank you and good luck!